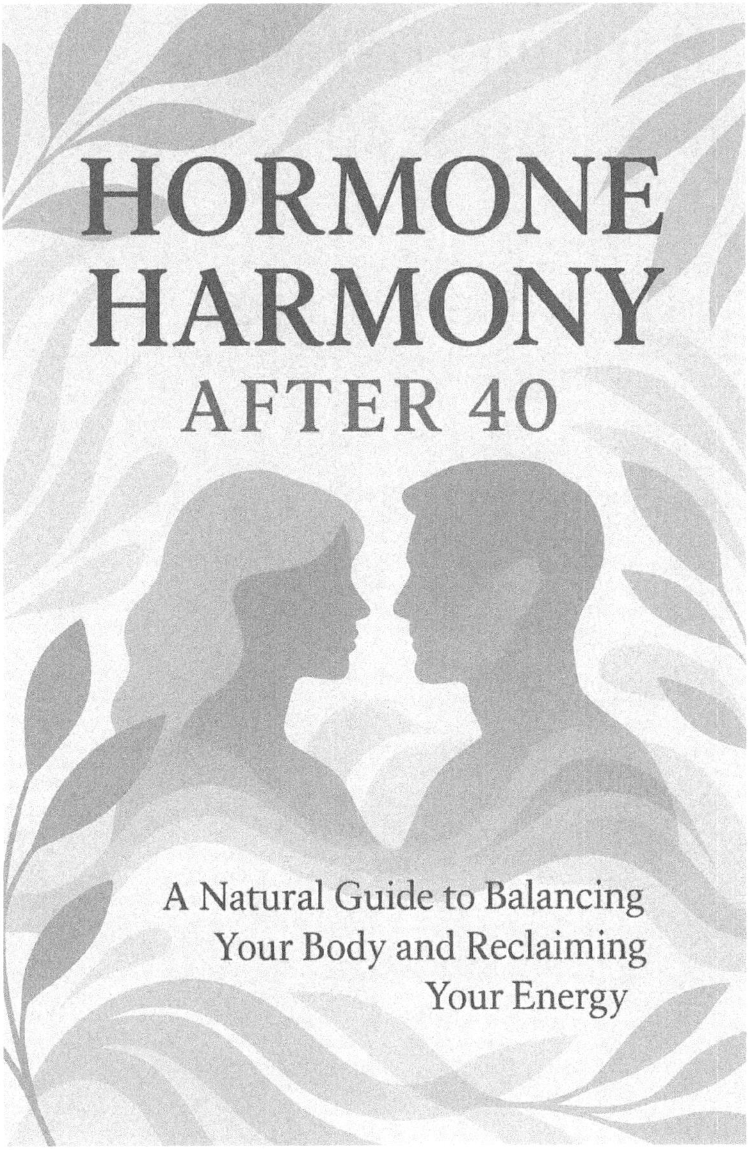
HORMONE
HARMONY
AFTER 40
A Natural Guide to Balancing
Your Body and Reclaiming
Your Energy

Hormone Harmony After 40

Dr. Mike Cockrell

ISBN:

Copyright © 2025

Medical Disclaimer

The information provided in this book is intended solely for educational and informational purposes. It is not intended as a substitute for professional medical advice, diagnosis, or treatment, nor should it be construed as such. The content reflects the author's opinions and research and is provided with the understanding that the author and publisher are not engaged in rendering medical, health, or other professional services.

Always seek the guidance of a qualified healthcare professional with any questions you may have regarding your health, medical conditions, or any changes you intend to make to your diet, lifestyle, supplement use, or exercise routine. Never disregard professional medical advice or delay in seeking it because of something you have read in this book.

Individual results may vary. The reader is solely responsible for their own health decisions, and any reliance on the information provided in this book is at their own risk. The author and publisher disclaim any liability for any adverse effects or consequences resulting from the use of any suggestions, recommendations, or procedures described herein.

If you are pregnant, nursing, taking medication, or have a medical condition, consult your physician or other qualified health provider before beginning any health-related program.

Contents

You're not crazy. You're not lazy. You're not just "getting older."

You're navigating the reality of hormonal changes—and for millions of men and women over 40, those changes can feel like a total body and mind hijack.

From sudden weight gain to unexplained fatigue, crashing libido, brain fog, anxiety, and sleep struggles—these symptoms are not just the "price of aging." They are messages from your body asking for support.

The good news? You *can* restore balance. And you don't always need harsh prescriptions to do it.

This book is your natural roadmap to understanding how your hormones shift after 40 and what you can do—safely and holistically—to bring your body back into harmony. You'll learn how to eat, move, supplement, and sleep in a way that supports your entire endocrine system.

Because when your hormones are happy, *you* are unstoppable.

For most of your life, your hormones have been silently working behind the scenes—regulating everything from energy, mood, metabolism, sleep, libido, and even your immune system. But once you hit your 40s, that quiet harmony often starts to shift. And for many people, it feels like everything starts changing at once.

But here's the truth: hormonal changes aren't just for women going through menopause. Men experience them too—through a less talked about but very real phenomenon called **andropause**. And both men and women need to understand how to support their bodies during this transitional phase, naturally and effectively.

The Shifting Landscape of Your 40s and Beyond

As you enter your 40s, the production of key hormones begins to decline—gradually in some, more rapidly in others. For women, this often marks the start of **perimenopause**, which can last for several years before menopause officially begins. During this time, estrogen and progesterone levels become erratic, causing symptoms like irritability, weight gain, night sweats, irregular cycles, and sleep disturbances.

For men, testosterone levels start to decline about 1% per year after the age of 30. By the time you're in your 40s or 50s, that can mean noticeable drops in muscle mass, energy, motivation, and sex drive—along with a rise in belly fat, fatigue, and even depression.

Symptoms You Shouldn't Ignore

If you're over 40 and experiencing any of the following, your hormones could be to blame:

- Low energy or motivation
- Difficulty sleeping or staying asleep
- Increased belly fat despite no major diet changes
- Brain fog or memory lapses
- Mood swings or irritability
- Loss of libido
- Irregular periods (for women)
- Hot flashes or night sweats
- Anxiety or a feeling of being "wired but tired"
- Hair thinning or changes in skin texture

These are not just random issues. They're warning signs that your endocrine system—the network of glands that produce your hormones—is out of sync.

Why This Matters More Than Ever

Unbalanced hormones don't just impact how you feel today. Over time, they can contribute to more serious conditions like:

- **Insulin resistance** and Type 2 diabetes
- **Osteoporosis** and loss of bone density
- **Cardiovascular disease**
- **Thyroid dysfunction**

- **Increased inflammation** and autoimmune flare-ups

The good news? Hormones are highly responsive to lifestyle changes. That means small, strategic shifts in your **nutrition, sleep, stress management, movement, and supplementation** can yield powerful results.

This Book is About Taking Control

You don't have to suffer through this chapter of life feeling depleted, discouraged, or disconnected from your body. By understanding how your hormones work—and what they need to thrive—you can restore balance, reclaim your energy, and feel like yourself again.

In the chapters ahead, we'll break down exactly how to do that.

Because hormonal health isn't a luxury—it's a necessity.

Before you can rebalance your hormones, you need to know what they are, what they do, and how they interact with each other. Hormones are your body's internal messengers—chemical signals that coordinate a wide range of essential functions. But when just one of them falls out of balance, the entire system can go haywire.

Let's break down the most important hormones for men and women over 40, how they function, and what happens when they're out of sync.

---

1. Estrogen (Primarily Female, But Men Have It Too)

What it does:
Estrogen regulates the female reproductive system, mood, bone density, and skin elasticity. In men, it supports libido, heart health, and brain function in small amounts.

What imbalance looks like:

- *Too low:* Hot flashes, vaginal dryness, mood swings, poor sleep, bone loss
- *Too high:* Weight gain (especially hips/thighs), mood swings, heavy periods, breast tenderness

Over 40 tip: Estrogen levels can spike and crash during perimenopause before dropping steadily after menopause. Supporting the liver and gut helps your body eliminate excess estrogen and restore balance.

---

2. Progesterone (The Calming Hormone)

What it does:
Known for its soothing, balancing effects, progesterone helps regulate mood, sleep, and menstrual cycles. It also supports fertility and counters the effects of estrogen.

What imbalance looks like:

- *Too low:* Anxiety, irritability, insomnia, short cycles, spotting, difficulty sleeping
- *Too high:* Rare, but could cause sleepiness or bloating

Over 40 tip: Stress lowers progesterone levels dramatically. Managing cortisol (your stress hormone) is key to restoring progesterone naturally.

---

3. Testosterone (Primarily Male, But Women Have It Too)

What it does:
Testosterone fuels energy, confidence, muscle mass, sex drive, and motivation. In women, it supports libido, metabolism, and mental clarity.

What imbalance looks like:

- *Too low:* Fatigue, low sex drive, loss of muscle, increased fat (especially around the midsection), brain fog, depression
- *Too high (in women):* Acne, facial hair, irregular periods, PCOS symptoms

Over 40 tip: Strength training, quality sleep, and zinc-rich foods can help naturally support testosterone levels.

---

4. Cortisol (The Stress Hormone)

What it does:
Cortisol is released in response to stress and helps regulate metabolism, blood sugar, inflammation, and immune responses. It's essential in small amounts, but damaging when chronically elevated.

What imbalance looks like:

- *Too high:* Belly fat, anxiety, poor sleep, sugar cravings, feeling "wired but tired"
- *Too low:* Burnout, low blood pressure, extreme fatigue, brain fog

Over 40 tip: Chronic stress is the fastest way to disrupt hormonal harmony. Breathwork, adaptogens, and proper rest are crucial to keeping cortisol balanced.

---

5. Insulin (The Blood Sugar Regulator)

What it does:
Insulin helps move sugar from your blood into your cells to use for energy. It works closely with cortisol and other hormones.

What imbalance looks like:

- *Too high (insulin resistance):* Belly fat, fatigue, cravings, brain fog, difficulty losing weight
- *Too low (hypoglycemia):* Shakiness, irritability, dizziness, hunger

Over 40 tip: As we age, our cells become less sensitive to insulin. A whole-foods, lower-glycemic diet and strength training can help improve insulin sensitivity.

---

6. Thyroid Hormones (T3 & T4)

What they do:
These hormones control metabolism, energy production, temperature regulation, and brain function. They are regulated by TSH (thyroid-stimulating hormone) from the pituitary gland.

What imbalance looks like:

- *Too low (hypothyroidism):* Fatigue, cold hands/feet, constipation, weight gain, depression, hair thinning
- *Too high (hyperthyroidism):* Anxiety, heart palpitations, weight loss, sweating, irritability

Over 40 tip: Thyroid function can slow down due to stress, nutrient deficiencies (especially iodine, selenium, zinc), or autoimmune conditions. Testing and targeted support can make a huge difference.

---

7. DHEA (The Mother Hormone)

What it does:
DHEA is a precursor to both testosterone and estrogen. It supports mood, libido, bone health, and energy.

What imbalance looks like:

- *Too low:* Low libido, fatigue, mood swings, reduced resilience to stress
- *Too high:* Acne, irritability, unwanted hair growth (in women)

Over 40 tip: DHEA naturally declines with age. Certain supplements may help, but consult a provider before using them long-term.

How These Hormones Work Together

Hormones don't operate in isolation. Think of them like members of a band—when one is off key, the whole performance suffers. For example:

- Elevated cortisol suppresses progesterone and thyroid function
- Insulin resistance affects testosterone and estrogen balance
- Low thyroid hormones can worsen estrogen dominance symptoms

That's why true hormone balance comes from a *whole-body* approach—not just treating one hormone at a time.

Key Takeaway: Know Your Hormones, Know Your Power

Understanding these hormonal players helps you make smarter choices about how you eat, sleep, move, and supplement. The rest of this guide will show you how to support them—naturally and safely—so you can feel strong, focused, and vibrant again.

Chapter 3: Hormonal Shifts in Women – From Perimenopause to Postmenopause

For many women, the decade of your 40s brings unexpected changes—not just physically, but emotionally and mentally. One day you might feel "off," and the next, you're dealing with hot flashes, unpredictable cycles, sudden anxiety, or weight gain around your midsection.

What's happening? The answer often lies in **hormonal shifts** associated with **perimenopause** and **menopause.**

This chapter breaks down what's going on inside your body, what symptoms to watch for, and most importantly—how to support yourself naturally through the process.

Understanding the Stages: Perimenopause, Menopause & Postmenopause

Perimenopause

This is the transitional phase before menopause. It can begin in your late 30s or early 40s and last anywhere from 2 to 10 years. During this time, your ovaries start producing less estrogen and progesterone, but not in a steady decline—it's more like a hormonal rollercoaster.

Common symptoms:

- Irregular periods (longer, shorter, heavier, or skipped)
- Mood swings, irritability, or anxiety
- Night sweats and hot flashes
- Sleep disturbances
- Decreased libido

- Brain fog or forgetfulness
- Breast tenderness
- Vaginal dryness
- Fatigue

Menopause
You officially reach menopause when you've gone 12 consecutive months without a menstrual cycle. The average age is around **51**, but it can happen earlier or later depending on genetics, lifestyle, or medical history.

At this stage, estrogen and progesterone levels drop significantly, and your reproductive years come to an end.

Postmenopause
This is the phase after menopause. While some symptoms may ease, others—like vaginal dryness, bone loss, or a slower metabolism—can persist or intensify.

What's Really Going On With Your Hormones

Here's a simplified look at what's happening:

- **Progesterone** drops first and faster than estrogen, often leading to **estrogen dominance**, which triggers bloating, mood swings, and heavy periods.
- **Estrogen** eventually begins to decline as well, leading to hot flashes, night sweats, and dryness.
- **Testosterone** also decreases, affecting libido, energy, and mental sharpness.
- **Cortisol and insulin** may become dysregulated due to stress and poor sleep, amplifying weight gain and fatigue.

In other words, your entire endocrine system is adapting—and sometimes struggling.

How Hormonal Shifts Affect Your Body

These changes can influence nearly every system in your body:

- **Weight and metabolism:** Hormonal shifts often slow metabolism and increase insulin resistance, leading to stubborn belly fat.
- **Brain and mood:** Estrogen plays a key role in serotonin production, so its decline can contribute to anxiety, depression, and memory issues.
- **Sleep:** Low progesterone (a calming hormone) can make it harder to fall and stay asleep.
- **Heart health:** Estrogen protects the cardiovascular system—its decline increases the risk of heart disease.
- **Bones and joints:** Estrogen also helps maintain bone density. Without it, women become more vulnerable to osteoporosis.
- **Sexual health:** Vaginal dryness, reduced libido, and painful intercourse are common, but treatable.

Natural Ways to Support Your Body Through the Transition

You don't need to white-knuckle your way through perimenopause or menopause. Natural strategies can dramatically improve how you feel.

1. Support Your Adrenals

The adrenal glands take over hormone production as the ovaries

slow down. When you're constantly stressed, they can't keep up.
Support strategies:

- Deep breathing or meditation
- Adaptogens like ashwagandha or rhodiola
- Consistent sleep and gentle movement

2. Balance Blood Sugar
Stable blood sugar supports cortisol and insulin regulation, which in turn helps estrogen and progesterone.
Support strategies:

- Eat protein, fat, and fiber at every meal
- Avoid refined carbs and sugars
- Don't skip meals

3. Prioritize Sleep
Sleep is when hormones reset.
Support strategies:

- Magnesium before bed
- Limit screens 1 hour before sleep
- Keep your bedroom cool and dark

4. Choose Hormone-Supportive Foods

- Cruciferous vegetables (broccoli, kale) help detox excess estrogen
- Omega-3s support inflammation and brain health
- Seeds like flax, pumpkin, and sesame can support natural hormone rhythms (*aka seed cycling*)

5. Move Your Body Wisely
Too much cardio can spike cortisol. Instead:

- Prioritize strength training
- Add in yoga or Pilates
- Go for daily walks

6. Supplement Intentionally

- **Magnesium** – supports sleep and hormone detox
- **Vitamin D** – essential for hormone production and mood
- **B-complex vitamins** – nourish the adrenals
- **Evening primrose oil or black cohosh** – help ease perimenopausal symptoms
- **Probiotics** – support gut health and hormone elimination

When to Seek Help

You don't need to suffer in silence. If your symptoms are severely impacting your life, seek out a provider who specializes in **functional medicine, integrative health, or hormone therapy.** Saliva or DUTCH hormone testing can help provide a full picture.

Key Takeaway: You're Not Broken—You're Evolving

Perimenopause and menopause are not diseases—they're transitions. But how you support your body through the shift can determine whether you feel empowered or exhausted.

With the right lifestyle shifts and natural support, you can thrive—not just survive—this next phase of life.

Chapter 4: Hormonal Changes in Men – Andropause and Beyond

Hormonal changes aren't just a "women's issue." Men experience a significant hormonal shift as they age too—only it happens more gradually and is often overlooked or misunderstood. This phase of male aging is sometimes referred to as **andropause**, or more commonly, **Low T (low testosterone)**.

But it's not just about testosterone.

Multiple hormones begin to shift for men after 40, and these changes can quietly impact energy, mood, motivation, body composition, sleep, sexual health, and even emotional resilience.

Let's break down what's really happening and how to naturally support your hormonal health as a man over 40.

What Is Andropause?

Andropause refers to the age-related decline in testosterone and other hormones in men, typically beginning around age 40 and continuing steadily each year.

Unlike menopause in women, which happens in a relatively short time span, andropause is gradual. Many men don't realize it's happening until the symptoms are affecting their quality of life.

Common Symptoms of Hormonal Changes in Men Over 40

- Low energy or chronic fatigue
- Reduced sex drive or erectile difficulties

- Depression, irritability, or emotional flatness
- Muscle loss and increased body fat, especially around the midsection
- Decreased strength or recovery time from workouts
- Difficulty concentrating or memory lapses
- Poor sleep or waking up unrefreshed
- Reduced motivation or "drive"

These symptoms aren't just the result of aging—they are red flags that your hormones, especially testosterone, may be out of balance.

Key Hormones Impacting Men's Health After 40

1. Testosterone (T)

- *Function:* Builds muscle, supports libido, drives motivation, supports red blood cell production, and enhances mental clarity.
- *What happens with age:* Production naturally drops about 1% per year after 30. Lifestyle stress, alcohol, insulin resistance, and sleep issues can accelerate that decline.
- *Imbalance signs:* Fatigue, loss of drive, low sex drive, depression, muscle weakness, and abdominal fat.

2. DHEA

- *Function:* A precursor hormone that helps produce testosterone and other androgens.
- *What happens with age:* Levels decline with aging and chronic stress.

- *Imbalance signs:* Low energy, mood issues, reduced resilience to stress.

3. Cortisol

- *Function:* The body's stress hormone. When balanced, it helps with energy and focus. When elevated chronically, it causes hormonal chaos.
- *Imbalance signs:* Belly fat, anxiety, poor sleep, burnout, low testosterone.

4. Insulin

- *Function:* Regulates blood sugar and energy.
- *Imbalance signs:* Fat gain (especially belly), fatigue, cravings, and increased risk for type 2 diabetes.

5. Estrogen (Yes, Men Have It Too!)

- *Function:* In small amounts, estrogen helps with brain function and libido.
- *What happens:* As testosterone declines, estrogen can become dominant—especially with poor liver function or excess body fat.
- *Imbalance signs:* Fat gain, mood swings, gynecomastia (male breast tissue), irritability.

Root Causes of Hormonal Decline in Men

- **Chronic stress** – suppresses testosterone and raises cortisol
- **Poor sleep** – one of the most overlooked causes of Low T

- **Sedentary lifestyle** – lowers testosterone and raises estrogen
- **Excess alcohol** – impairs liver detox, raising estrogen
- **High sugar/carb intake** – causes insulin resistance
- **Environmental toxins** – plastics, pesticides, and chemicals disrupt hormone function

How to Naturally Support Hormonal Health After 40

You can take powerful, natural steps to support your body's hormone production and regulation.

1. Prioritize Strength Training

- Builds lean muscle and boosts testosterone
- Short, intense sessions (30–45 minutes) are ideal
- Focus on compound movements: squats, deadlifts, pushups, rows

2. Optimize Sleep Quality

- Aim for 7–8 hours in a dark, cool room
- Avoid screens and blue light before bed
- Supplement with magnesium or L-theanine if needed

3. Eat Testosterone-Friendly Foods

- Zinc-rich foods (oysters, pumpkin seeds, grass-fed beef)
- Healthy fats (avocados, olive oil, wild salmon)
- Cruciferous vegetables (broccoli, cauliflower) to reduce excess estrogen

- Avoid soy, alcohol, and ultra-processed foods

4. Lower Your Stress Load

- Practice breathwork, meditation, or mindfulness
- Add adaptogens like ashwagandha, rhodiola, or maca
- Prioritize downtime and creative outlets

5. Maintain a Healthy Weight

- Visceral fat (belly fat) converts testosterone into estrogen
- Losing even 10–15 pounds can dramatically improve hormonal balance

6. Use Targeted Supplementation

- **Vitamin D** – boosts testosterone and immune function
- **Zinc and magnesium** – support testosterone production and stress response
- **Omega-3s** – reduce inflammation and support brain health
- **DHEA (if tested low)** – may be appropriate under supervision

Testing and Monitoring Your Hormones

If you suspect low testosterone or other hormonal imbalances, it's worth getting tested.

Tests to consider:

- Total and Free Testosterone
- Estradiol

- DHEA-S
- Cortisol (saliva or DUTCH test)
- Fasting insulin and glucose
- SHBG (sex hormone-binding globulin)

Work with a hormone-literate healthcare provider who can interpret these results and help you build a personalized support plan.

Key Takeaway: Hormonal Health Is Vital for a Thriving Life After 40

You don't have to accept fatigue, weight gain, low libido, or loss of motivation as your "new normal."

With strategic lifestyle changes and natural support, you can maintain strong testosterone levels, sharp mental focus, emotional stability, and a powerful sense of vitality—well into your 50s, 60s, and beyond.

Chapter 5: Top Signs of Hormonal Imbalance (and What to Do About Them)

You're dragging through the day with no energy… snapping at people you love… gaining weight for no obvious reason… or lying awake at night even though you're exhausted.

If any of that sounds familiar, your hormones could be out of balance.

Hormonal imbalances often go undiagnosed because the symptoms are subtle, gradual, and easy to dismiss as "normal aging" or "stress." But your body is constantly sending signals—and when hormones are off, those signals get louder.

This chapter breaks down the most common signs of hormonal imbalance and what they actually mean—plus simple, natural ways to start restoring harmony.

1. Chronic Fatigue

You're getting 7–8 hours of sleep, but still feel wiped out by midday. This isn't normal—it's a red flag.

What's going on:

- Low thyroid function
- Adrenal dysfunction (high or low cortisol)
- Low testosterone or estrogen
- Blood sugar instability due to insulin resistance

What to do:

- Prioritize deep sleep (consistent bedtime, no screens before bed)
- Eat more protein and fewer refined carbs
- Support your adrenals with adaptogens like ashwagandha
- Get tested for thyroid, testosterone, and cortisol levels

2. Weight Gain—Especially Around the Belly

You haven't changed your diet, but your jeans don't fit anymore—especially around the waist.

What's going on:

- Elevated cortisol from chronic stress
- Estrogen dominance or testosterone decline
- Insulin resistance

What to do:

- Cut sugar and refined carbs
- Add daily movement (walking + strength training)
- Support liver detox with cruciferous vegetables
- Manage stress (deep breathing, meditation, adaptogens)

3. Mood Swings, Anxiety, or Depression

One minute you're fine, the next you're snapping at your spouse or spiraling in anxiety.

What's going on:

- Estrogen/progesterone imbalance (especially in women)
- Low testosterone (in men and women)
- Blood sugar crashes
- Low thyroid function

What to do:

- Eat protein every 3–4 hours to stabilize blood sugar
- Get sunlight in the morning to support cortisol rhythm
- Try magnesium or L-theanine for natural calming support
- Track your cycle (women) or mood patterns (men) and correlate with symptoms

4. Brain Fog or Memory Issues

You forget where you put your keys, why you walked into the room, or what someone just said.

What's going on:

- Low estrogen or testosterone
- Insulin resistance (blood sugar rollercoasters)
- High cortisol and poor sleep
- Thyroid dysfunction

What to do:

- Eat omega-3s daily (wild salmon, walnuts, fish oil)
- Reduce multitasking and digital overload

- Balance blood sugar with whole foods
- Get 7–9 hours of restorative sleep

5. Low Libido

You love your partner, but the drive just isn't there—and hasn't been for a while.

What's going on:

- Low testosterone or DHEA (in both men and women)
- Estrogen imbalance (in women)
- High cortisol
- Poor blood flow and inflammation

What to do:

- Lift weights to naturally boost testosterone
- Add maca or tribulus to your routine
- Eat circulation-supporting foods (beets, pomegranate, leafy greens)
- Cut alcohol and increase hydration

6. Sleep Problems

You can't fall asleep, stay asleep, or feel rested in the morning.

What's going on:

- Low progesterone (in women)
- High cortisol at night

- Blood sugar drops during sleep
- Low melatonin or magnesium

What to do:

- Stop eating 2–3 hours before bed
- Create a wind-down routine: magnesium, herbal tea, no screens
- Try adaptogens or calming teas in the evening (like chamomile or lemon balm)
- Keep your bedroom cool and dark

7. Digestive Issues

You're bloated, constipated, or dealing with gas or indigestion—even when you eat "healthy."

What's going on:

- Estrogen imbalance affecting bile production
- Cortisol shutting down digestion during stress
- Low thyroid slowing gut motility
- Gut dysbiosis impacting hormone detox

What to do:

- Add probiotics and fiber-rich foods
- Eat slowly and chew thoroughly
- Reduce caffeine and alcohol
- Consider digestive enzymes or bitters before meals

8. Irregular Periods or Menstrual Changes (Women)

Your cycle is all over the place—longer, shorter, heavier, or missing altogether.

What's going on:

- Perimenopause (fluctuating estrogen and progesterone)
- Estrogen dominance
- Thyroid dysfunction
- Blood sugar imbalance

What to do:

- Track your cycle for 2–3 months
- Support liver detox and progesterone with seed cycling
- Try chasteberry (vitex) or evening primrose oil
- Balance blood sugar to reduce PMS and inflammation

9. Loss of Muscle and Strength

You're working out, but can't build muscle—or you're losing it faster than ever.

What's going on:

- Declining testosterone and growth hormone
- Chronic inflammation or cortisol elevation
- Low protein intake or poor nutrient absorption

What to do:

- Strength train 3x per week
- Get at least 100g of high-quality protein daily
- Consider amino acid supplementation
- Sleep 7–9 hours to support recovery and growth

10. Thinning Hair or Dry Skin

Your hair feels thinner, your nails brittle, and your skin dry or dull.

What's going on:

- Low thyroid hormone
- Estrogen or progesterone decline
- Poor nutrient absorption (especially zinc, biotin, iron, omega-3s)

What to do:

- Test your thyroid (especially free T3 and T4)
- Increase omega-3 intake
- Add collagen or silica supplements
- Hydrate and use toxin-free skincare

When Should You Get Tested?

If you're experiencing multiple symptoms, it's worth running comprehensive hormone tests. Look for a provider who can help you order:

- Cortisol (saliva or DUTCH test)
- Estradiol, progesterone, testosterone
- DHEA-S
- Thyroid panel (TSH, Free T3, Free T4, Reverse T3)
- Fasting insulin, glucose, HbA1c
- SHBG (sex hormone binding globulin)

Key Takeaway: Listen to the Whispers Before They Become Screams

Your body is always communicating with you. If you're feeling "off," that's not something to ignore—it's something to investigate.

In the next chapters, we'll explore natural tools you can use to bring your hormones back into alignment—so you can stop surviving and start thriving again.

Hormonal health is not just about age or genetics—it's deeply connected to the way you live your life every single day.

What you eat, how you move, how much stress you carry, how well you sleep, and even your exposure to toxins can either **nurture your hormones or sabotage them**.

If you're over 40 and noticing signs of imbalance, it's time to look beyond symptom management and dive into the root cause: your **daily habits**.

This chapter reveals the powerful, science-backed connection between your lifestyle and hormone function—and shows you how to make simple adjustments that can create big changes.

Your Daily Choices Shape Your Hormones

Hormones don't just "decline with age"—they decline faster when they're under attack from modern living.

Think of your hormones like a team of high-performing athletes. If they're fueled with junk, pushed too hard, and never allowed to rest, they can't perform. But with the right support, they can thrive—even after 40.

Here are the five most critical lifestyle factors that directly influence hormonal health:

1. Nutrition: Food Is Information for Your Hormones

Everything you eat sends messages to your body—either to promote balance or create chaos.

The problem:

- Highly processed foods, refined carbs, sugar, and inflammatory oils spike insulin and cortisol
- Excess caffeine and alcohol deplete key hormone-supportive nutrients
- Low protein intake can weaken muscle and lower testosterone

The solution:

- Eat *real, whole foods*—especially protein, fiber, healthy fats, and colorful vegetables
- Focus on *blood sugar balance*: every meal should contain protein, fat, and fiber
- Support liver detox with cruciferous vegetables (broccoli, kale, cauliflower, Brussels sprouts)
- Hydrate well—dehydration can impair every hormonal process

2. Stress: The Hormone Disruptor You Can't Ignore

Chronic stress is one of the most powerful disruptors of hormonal balance. When stress is high, your body floods with cortisol—and when cortisol is elevated long-term, it depletes sex hormones like estrogen, progesterone, and testosterone.

The problem:

- Your body can't tell the difference between a looming deadline and an actual life-or-death threat
- Stress hormones shut down reproductive, digestive, and thyroid function to prioritize survival

The solution:

- Start your day with calming rituals—meditation, journaling, stretching
- Schedule "white space" into your day (time with no obligations)
- Practice deep breathing or box breathing (inhale for 4, hold for 4, exhale for 4, hold for 4)
- Try calming adaptogens like ashwagandha, holy basil, or rhodiola

3. Sleep: The Time When Hormones Reset

Your hormones repair, rebuild, and rebalance while you sleep—especially during deep and REM stages.

The problem:

- Blue light, late-night snacks, alcohol, and inconsistent sleep patterns disrupt melatonin and cortisol rhythms
- Poor sleep raises ghrelin (hunger hormone) and lowers leptin (fullness hormone), which contributes to weight gain

The solution:

- Create a consistent bedtime routine and aim for 7–9 hours of uninterrupted sleep
- Shut down screens at least one hour before bed
- Keep your room cool, dark, and quiet
- Supplement with magnesium glycinate or L-theanine if needed

4. Movement: Exercise for Hormone Optimization

Exercise isn't just about burning calories—it's one of the most effective tools for hormonal balance.

The problem:

- Too much high-intensity cardio can raise cortisol and break down muscle
- Too little movement reduces testosterone, insulin sensitivity, and metabolism

The solution:

- Strength training 2–4 times per week supports testosterone and growth hormone
- Walking 30 minutes a day lowers cortisol and improves insulin sensitivity
- Gentle movement (yoga, Pilates, stretching) supports lymph flow and reduces inflammation

5. Toxin Exposure: The Hidden Hormone Saboteurs

Many modern products contain **endocrine disruptors**—chemicals that mimic or block hormones and interfere with your endocrine system.

The problem:

- BPA, phthalates, parabens, and pesticides are everywhere: in plastics, skincare, cleaning supplies, and even food packaging

- These toxins can mimic estrogen (leading to estrogen dominance), reduce testosterone, and overload your liver

The solution:

- Use glass or stainless steel instead of plastic for food and water
- Switch to non-toxic cleaning and personal care products (look for "fragrance-free" or "EWG Verified")
- Eat organic when possible—especially for the "Dirty Dozen" fruits and vegetables
- Support your detox organs (liver, kidneys, lymph) with hydration, sweating, and fiber-rich foods

Lifestyle Isn't Just Prevention—It's Power

By making hormone-smart lifestyle choices, you give your body the foundation it needs to regulate hormones naturally, heal imbalances, and restore optimal function.

Even small changes—like getting to bed 30 minutes earlier, adding 15 minutes of daily walking, or switching to a clean skincare line—can add up to big results.

Key Takeaway: Your Daily Routine Is Either Balancing Your Hormones or Breaking Them Down

You don't need to overhaul your entire life overnight. But you *do* need to start somewhere.

In the next chapters, we'll break down how to eat, supplement, and move to support hormone harmony in a natural, sustainable way—starting with **Chapter 7: Nutrition for Hormonal Balance**.

You've probably heard the phrase "food is medicine," but when it comes to your hormones, food is also *information*.

Every bite you take sends signals to your endocrine system. It tells your body whether to burn fat or store it, whether to make sex hormones or stress hormones, and whether to calm inflammation or amplify it.

And after 40, your nutritional needs shift—what worked in your 20s or 30s may no longer serve your body today.

This chapter is your guide to eating in a way that supports hormone production, detoxification, and balance—naturally and sustainably.

The Three Pillars of Hormone-Supportive Nutrition

1. **Balance Blood Sugar**
2. **Reduce Inflammation**
3. **Support Detoxification**

Let's break each one down.

1. Balance Blood Sugar to Balance Hormones

When your blood sugar is unstable, your body produces more insulin to compensate. Over time, this leads to **insulin resistance**, which disrupts cortisol, estrogen, testosterone, and thyroid hormones.

Symptoms of blood sugar imbalance:

- Energy crashes
- Cravings (especially for sugar or carbs)
- Weight gain around the belly
- Irritability or "hanger"
- Brain fog

Daily strategies to balance blood sugar:

- Eat **protein at every meal** (aim for 20–30g)
- Include **healthy fats** (avocado, olive oil, nuts, seeds)
- Add **fiber** (leafy greens, berries, legumes) to slow glucose spikes
- Avoid skipping meals—this can trigger cortisol spikes
- Limit refined sugar, white flour, and processed snacks

Pro tip: Start your day with a high-protein breakfast (like eggs, turkey sausage, or a clean protein shake)—this sets the tone for balanced energy and hormones all day.

2. Reduce Inflammation to Unclog Hormonal Pathways

Chronic inflammation is at the root of nearly every hormone imbalance. It blocks communication between your glands and can suppress hormone production.

Top inflammatory foods to avoid or minimize:

- Refined sugar and high-fructose corn syrup
- Industrial seed oils (canola, soybean, corn oil)
- Excess alcohol

- Ultra-processed snacks and convenience meals
- Artificial sweeteners and food dyes

Anti-inflammatory foods to add in daily:

- Wild salmon, sardines, or omega-3 supplements
- Leafy greens like kale, spinach, and arugula
- Berries (blueberries, raspberries, blackberries)
- Turmeric, ginger, cinnamon, and garlic
- Bone broth and collagen-rich foods

3. Support Detoxification to Clear Hormonal Waste

Your body must **break down and eliminate old hormones**—especially estrogen—every single day. If your liver, gut, or lymphatic system is sluggish, hormones build up and recirculate, creating imbalances.

Key detox-supporting nutrients and foods:

- **Cruciferous vegetables**: broccoli, cauliflower, Brussels sprouts, kale
- **Lemon water**: stimulates liver enzymes
- **Fiber**: found in chia seeds, flax, oats, lentils, beans
- **Green tea**: supports liver enzymes and antioxidants
- **Beets and carrots**: help cleanse the liver and support bile flow

Pro tip: Include a daily green smoothie with leafy greens, lemon, flaxseed, and clean protein for an easy hormone-loving detox boost.

Superfoods for Hormonal Health

Here's a list of superstar foods that nourish your endocrine system:

Food	Hormonal Benefit
Pumpkin seeds	Rich in zinc – supports testosterone and immune health
Avocados	Healthy fats that build hormones and reduce inflammation
Flaxseeds	Contains lignans that help balance estrogen
Maca root	Adaptogen that may boost libido and energy
Wild-caught salmon	Rich in omega-3s for hormone and brain health
Eggs	Provide cholesterol, the building block of steroid hormones
Berries	Antioxidants that fight inflammation and support hormone regulation
Leafy greens	Provide magnesium, folate, and fiber for detox and balance
Fermented foods (sauerkraut, kimchi, kefir)	Feed gut bacteria that help process and eliminate hormones

What About Coffee and Alcohol?

Coffee:

- In moderation, coffee can be beneficial, but overuse may increase cortisol.
- Limit to 1–2 cups/day, always with food—not on an empty stomach.
- Consider switching to matcha, herbal coffee alternatives, or half-caf blends if you're feeling anxious or wired.

Alcohol:

- Alcohol raises estrogen, disrupts liver detox, and depletes B vitamins.
- Limit to 1–2 drinks per week, and always hydrate well after.
- Choose cleaner options: dry red wine, tequila with soda water, or organic cider.

Sample Hormone-Friendly Daily Meal Plan

Breakfast

- 2 eggs + sautéed spinach + ½ avocado
- Side of berries
- Green tea or lemon water

Lunch

- Grilled salmon salad with arugula, roasted veggies, olive oil, and lemon
- Small handful of walnuts or pumpkin seeds

Snack

- Chia pudding with almond milk, flax, cinnamon, and berries
  or
- Protein smoothie with clean protein powder, leafy greens, flax, and almond butter

Dinner

- Grass-fed beef or turkey burger (no bun)
- Roasted sweet potatoes and broccoli
- Side of sauerkraut or fermented pickles

Optional Evening Calm Drink

- Herbal tea with magnesium or a calming adaptogen like reishi

Key Takeaway: Eat Like Your Hormones Are Listening—Because They Are

You don't need a restrictive diet to feel your best—you need a *strategic* one. Fueling your body with the right foods helps your hormones do what they're designed to do: keep you energized, focused, calm, and resilient.

Next up, we'll dive into **Chapter 8: The Power of Adaptogens and Herbal Support**—where you'll learn how nature's most powerful plants can help bring your hormones back into balance.

Chapter 8: The Power of Adaptogens and Herbal Support

What if there were natural, plant-based tools that could help your body adapt to stress, support hormonal balance, and restore energy—without relying on synthetic hormones or harsh medications?

Good news: there are. They're called **adaptogens**.

These powerful herbs and roots have been used for centuries in Ayurvedic, Chinese, and Indigenous medicine systems—and modern science is finally catching up. Adaptogens work by helping your body find equilibrium. Whether you're too wired, too tired, or hormonally out of whack, these botanical allies help you come back to center.

In this chapter, you'll learn how adaptogens and hormone-supportive herbs can help restore balance in your 40s and beyond—plus how to choose the right ones for your unique needs.

What Are Adaptogens?

Adaptogens are a unique class of herbs that:

- Help the body adapt to physical, mental, and emotional stress
- Normalize imbalances (rather than push hormones in one direction)
- Regulate cortisol and support adrenal health
- Enhance resilience, energy, and focus without overstimulation

Think of them as *intelligent plants*—they respond to what your body needs in the moment.

Top Adaptogens and Herbs for Hormonal Health

1. Ashwagandha *(Withania somnifera)*

Benefits:

- Reduces cortisol and anxiety
- Improves sleep quality
- Supports thyroid and adrenal function
- May increase testosterone in men and libido in women

Best for: Burnout, chronic stress, insomnia, low thyroid, mood swings
How to use: Powder, capsules, or tincture—often taken at night for calming effect

2. Rhodiola Rosea

Benefits:

- Increases stamina, mental clarity, and physical performance
- Balances cortisol (especially if it's too low in the morning)
- Supports mood and reduces fatigue

Best for: Low energy, mental fog, mild depression, sluggish mornings
How to use: Capsules or tincture—typically taken earlier in the day

3. Maca Root *(Lepidium meyenii)*

Benefits:

- Supports estrogen and testosterone balance
- Boosts libido and sexual function
- Enhances mood, energy, and fertility

Best for: Low libido, perimenopause, hormonal fatigue
How to use: Powder (in smoothies or oatmeal) or capsules—best taken in the morning

4. Holy Basil (Tulsi)

Benefits:

- Calms the nervous system
- Supports healthy cortisol levels
- Promotes emotional resilience
- Reduces blood sugar and inflammation

Best for: Anxiety, emotional stress, insulin resistance
How to use: Tea (delicious and calming), tincture, or capsules

5. Schisandra Berry

Benefits:

- Supports liver detoxification
- Balances estrogen metabolism

- Boosts skin health and endurance
- Enhances mental focus

Best for: Hormonal detox support, skin clarity, PMS, focus
How to use: Powder or tincture—great for morning use

6. Reishi Mushroom

Benefits:

- Deeply calming adaptogen
- Supports immune and adrenal function
- Enhances sleep and stress resilience
- Contains antioxidants that support hormone balance

Best for: Insomnia, chronic fatigue, immune health, menopause support
How to use: Capsules, powders, or nighttime tea blends

7. Vitex (Chasteberry) *(For women only)*

Benefits:

- Balances progesterone and reduces estrogen dominance
- Eases PMS and perimenopausal symptoms
- Regulates menstrual cycles

Best for: Irregular periods, mood swings, breast tenderness, hormonal acne
How to use: Capsules or tincture—best taken first thing in the morning

8. Tribulus Terrestris *(For men mostly)*

Benefits:

- Supports testosterone production
- Improves sexual function and stamina
- May help with muscle strength and recovery

Best for: Low libido, erectile challenges, muscle loss
How to use: Capsules—follow product dosing guidelines

How to Choose the Right Adaptogen

Your symptoms can help guide your selection. Here's a simple reference table:

Symptom / Goal	Best Adaptogens
Fatigue / Burnout	Ashwagandha, Rhodiola, Maca
Anxiety / Mood Swings	Holy Basil, Reishi, Ashwagandha
Poor Sleep	Reishi, Ashwagandha, Lemon Balm (non-adaptogen)
Hormonal Imbalance (Women)	Vitex, Maca, Schisandra
Low Testosterone / Libido (Men)	Tribulus, Maca, Ashwagandha
Menopause Support	Maca, Reishi, Schisandra

Symptom / Goal	Best Adaptogens
Estrogen Detox / PMS	Schisandra, Holy Basil, Vitex
Mental Focus / Brain Fog	Rhodiola, Schisandra, Lion's Mane (non-adaptogen)

How to Safely Use Adaptogens

- **Start slow:** Begin with one adaptogen at a time to see how your body responds.
- **Cycle them:** Use for 6–8 weeks, then take a short break to reset.
- **Pair with food:** Some herbs are best absorbed with meals (especially fat-soluble ones).
- **Watch for interactions:** If you're on medication or have thyroid/adrenal conditions, consult your provider.
- **Quality matters:** Choose organic, standardized extracts from reputable brands—avoid cheap or untested blends.

Bonus: Herbal Teas for Daily Hormone Support

Don't underestimate the power of a good tea blend! Try these:

- **Hormone Balance Tea:** Tulsi, red raspberry leaf, spearmint, nettle
- **Stress Soother:** Chamomile, ashwagandha, lavender
- **Liver Detox Tea:** Dandelion root, ginger, milk thistle
- **Sleep Support Tea:** Reishi, passionflower, lemon balm

Key Takeaway: Let Nature Help You Rebalance

Adaptogens are not quick fixes—but over time, they can gently and powerfully support your body's return to hormonal balance, especially when paired with proper nutrition, movement, and stress reduction.

They work *with* your body—not against it—making them an ideal solution for those navigating their 40s, 50s, and beyond.

Next up: **Chapter 9 – Gut Health and Hormones**, where we'll explore how your microbiome affects estrogen, mood, metabolism, and more.

You've probably heard that "the gut is the second brain," but here's something even more important—your gut is also one of your **biggest hormone regulators.**

Yes, your digestive system plays a powerful role in producing, converting, and eliminating hormones. In fact, if your gut is unhealthy, your hormones *can't* be balanced—no matter how clean you eat, how many supplements you take, or how well you sleep.

This chapter will show you the powerful connection between gut health and hormone balance—and how to heal your gut to support your hormones naturally.

The Gut-Hormone Superhighway

Your gut and hormones are in constant communication through:

1. **The Microbiome** – trillions of bacteria that help regulate metabolism, immunity, mood, and estrogen detox
2. **The Gut-Liver Axis** – your liver processes hormones, and your gut helps eliminate them
3. **The Estrobolome** – a specific collection of gut bacteria that metabolizes estrogen
4. **The Gut-Brain Axis** – your gut produces neurotransmitters like serotonin and dopamine, which influence mood and stress hormones

So when your gut is inflamed, leaky, or imbalanced, your hormones can go haywire too.

Signs Your Gut May Be Disrupting Your Hormones

- Bloating, gas, or constipation
- Sugar cravings or blood sugar crashes
- Skin issues (acne, eczema, rosacea)
- Mood swings, anxiety, or depression
- PMS or heavy periods
- Poor sleep or fatigue
- Food sensitivities or histamine issues
- Brain fog or low focus

These symptoms aren't "just gut problems"—they're **hormone problems rooted in your gut**.

The Gut and Estrogen Detox

Your liver filters out old, used-up estrogen from the body. But guess what? The estrogen can't leave *unless* your gut does its job to excrete it.

If you're constipated, eating too little fiber, or have an overgrowth of "bad" gut bacteria, that estrogen gets **reabsorbed** into your system—leading to **estrogen dominance**.

Symptoms of estrogen dominance:

- Heavy or painful periods
- Breast tenderness
- Mood swings or irritability
- Belly fat and bloating

- Fibroids or endometriosis

Leaky Gut and Inflammation: The Hormone Hijackers

When your gut lining becomes permeable (aka "leaky gut"), toxins and undigested food particles leak into your bloodstream. This triggers **inflammation** and overactivates your immune system, which can:

- Disrupt thyroid hormones
- Suppress progesterone
- Interfere with testosterone production
- Worsen insulin resistance

How to Heal Your Gut and Balance Your Hormones

Here's your gut-supportive, hormone-boosting game plan:

1. Feed the Good Bugs (Your Microbiome)

Add in fermented, fiber-rich, and prebiotic foods:

- Sauerkraut, kimchi, kefir, yogurt, miso
- Garlic, onions, leeks, asparagus, bananas
- Ground flaxseeds and chia seeds
- Apples, oats, lentils, and leafy greens

Tip: Aim for 30 different plant foods per week for microbiome diversity.

2. Remove the Gut Disruptors

Cut out the common culprits that inflame the gut:

- Refined sugar and processed foods
- Excess alcohol
- Gluten and dairy (if sensitive)
- Artificial sweeteners (especially sucralose, aspartame)
- NSAIDs and antibiotics (unless absolutely necessary)

Tip: Consider an elimination diet for 2–4 weeks if symptoms are severe.

3. Support Digestion

Your gut can't function well if you're rushing, stressed, or lacking stomach acid.

- Eat slowly and chew thoroughly
- Don't multitask during meals
- Try digestive bitters or enzymes before large meals
- Drink warm lemon water in the morning to stimulate digestion

Bonus: Apple cider vinegar before meals may help those with low stomach acid (start with 1 tsp in water).

4. Keep Things Moving

Daily bowel movements are essential for eliminating used-up hormones—especially estrogen.

- Aim for 25–35g of fiber per day
- Drink at least half your body weight in ounces of water
- Move your body daily (walking, yoga, strength training)
- Consider magnesium citrate if you're constipated

5. Add Probiotics and Gut-Healing Nutrients

Supplements to support your gut-hormone connection:

- **Probiotics:** Look for broad-spectrum formulas with Lactobacillus and Bifidobacterium strains
- **L-Glutamine:** Helps repair the gut lining
- **Zinc carnosine:** Reduces gut inflammation
- **Collagen peptides or bone broth:** Nourish the gut lining and reduce inflammation
- **Aloe vera juice (inner leaf):** Soothes irritated digestive tissues

6. Support Liver Detox (So Estrogen Doesn't Build Up)

- Eat cruciferous vegetables daily (broccoli, cabbage, cauliflower)
- Add lemon to your water
- Take a high-quality B-complex vitamin
- Include liver-supporting herbs like milk thistle, dandelion root, and turmeric

- Avoid excess alcohol and chemicals from conventional cleaning/personal care products

Gut Reset: A Sample Day of Eating for Gut & Hormone Health

Morning:

- Warm lemon water + probiotic
- Scrambled eggs with spinach and avocado
- 1 scoop collagen in herbal tea

Midday:

- Grilled chicken or salmon salad with olive oil, beets, carrots, and fermented pickles
- 1 tbsp ground flax in a smoothie or mixed into the salad

Afternoon snack:

- Chia pudding with cinnamon + berries
- Herbal tea (peppermint, ginger, or chamomile)

Dinner:

- Roasted vegetables with quinoa and turmeric tahini sauce
- Sautéed kale or cabbage
- Kefir or coconut yogurt for dessert (unsweetened)

Key Takeaway: Heal Your Gut, Heal Your Hormones

Your gut isn't just where food gets digested—it's where hormone health begins. A nourished, balanced gut leads to better estrogen clearance, steadier moods, more stable energy, and fewer symptoms across the board.

If you've been treating hormone symptoms but still feel "off," your gut might be the missing piece.

Next up: **Chapter 10 – Sleep, Stress, and Circadian Rhythm Repair**, where we'll look at how your sleep-wake cycle—and how well you manage stress—can either restore or wreck your hormonal balance.

Chapter 10: Sleep, Stress, and Circadian Rhythm Repair

If there were one "magic switch" for better hormone balance, it would be **restorative sleep** and a healthy stress response.

In your 40s and beyond, your hormones are more sensitive to two major disruptors: **chronic stress** and **poor sleep hygiene**. Both have the power to completely derail your endocrine system—raising cortisol, lowering testosterone, throwing off estrogen and progesterone, and suppressing thyroid function.

This chapter is all about restoring your natural rhythms so your body can return to balance, regenerate overnight, and handle stress like a champ.

How Stress Impacts Your Hormones

Stress is not just emotional—it's hormonal.

When you're under stress (even the low-grade kind like emails, traffic, or late-night scrolling), your adrenal glands release **cortisol** to help you "survive." That's great short-term. But when stress is constant, cortisol stays elevated, and your body enters a state of hormonal imbalance.

Chronic high cortisol causes:

- Fat storage (especially around the belly)
- Blood sugar spikes and insulin resistance
- Suppressed thyroid function
- Low progesterone (leading to estrogen dominance)
- Low testosterone and DHEA
- Poor sleep and mood regulation

Even worse? Your body prioritizes survival over everything else. That means your reproductive, metabolic, and digestive systems take a back seat.

How Sleep Regulates Hormones

Sleep is your body's nightly hormone reset. It's when:

- Cortisol drops so melatonin (your sleep hormone) can rise
- Growth hormone is released (for muscle repair and fat burning)
- Your liver detoxes hormones like estrogen
- Leptin and ghrelin (hunger hormones) rebalance
- Testosterone and progesterone are restored

But if you're tossing, turning, or staying up late, this critical cycle is disrupted—especially after 40, when melatonin naturally declines.

Signs You're Stuck in a Hormonal Stress Loop

- You feel tired but wired at night
- You wake up between 2–4 a.m. with anxiety
- You crash after lunch
- You crave carbs, sugar, or salt
- You feel overwhelmed by small things
- You can't sleep even though you're exhausted

- You wake up feeling unrested no matter how early you went to bed

How to Reset Your Stress + Sleep Rhythms Naturally

□ Daytime Strategies for Cortisol Balance

1. Get morning sunlight

- 10–20 minutes within 30–60 minutes of waking
- Regulates your cortisol-melatonin rhythm
- Boosts mood and metabolism

2. Eat breakfast with protein and fat

- Keeps blood sugar stable and prevents cortisol spikes
- Examples: eggs + avocado, protein smoothie, turkey sausage + sautéed spinach

3. Move your body (but don't overtrain)

- Walking, light cardio, yoga, or strength training all help lower cortisol
- Too much high-intensity exercise can spike it

4. Practice "mini stress resets" throughout the day

- Deep belly breathing
- 5-minute walk outdoors
- Mindfulness or prayer breaks
- Box breathing or alternate nostril breathing

5. Avoid stimulants after 2 p.m.

- Caffeine too late in the day disrupts melatonin production
- Try herbal adaptogenic teas instead (holy basil, rooibos, chamomile)

☽ Evening Strategies for Melatonin + Recovery Hormones

1. Create a wind-down routine

- No screens 60 minutes before bed
- Dim the lights after sunset
- Use blue light blocking glasses
- Journaling or a calming book helps shift your brain into "rest mode"

2. Support your nervous system

- Take **magnesium glycinate** or **L-theanine**
- Drink calming herbal teas (chamomile, lemon balm, passionflower)
- Epsom salt baths soothe both muscles and your mind

3. Keep your sleep environment sacred

- Cool room (65–68°F)
- Total darkness (use blackout curtains or an eye mask)
- White noise machine or fan
- No phones or TVs in the bedroom

4. Eat to support sleep (but not too late)

- Light, balanced dinner 2–3 hours before bed
- Avoid heavy meals, sugar, or alcohol
- Small sleep snack: banana with almond butter or herbal tea with a collagen peptide

Supplements to Support Circadian and Adrenal Rhythm

Supplement	Benefits
Magnesium Glycinate	Calms the nervous system, improves sleep depth
Ashwagandha	Regulates cortisol, helps with stress resilience
Rhodiola	Supports adrenal health and morning energy
Phosphatidylserine	Helps lower nighttime cortisol
L-theanine	Promotes relaxation without sedation
Reishi Mushroom	Enhances immune and sleep cycles
Melatonin (short term)	Helps reestablish rhythm, especially during transitions

Note: Always check with your healthcare provider before starting new supplements, especially if you're taking medications.

Bonus Practice: The Power of Breath for Hormone Reset

When stress hits, your breath becomes shallow and rapid—triggering more cortisol. Reversing that pattern with conscious breath work can instantly shift your nervous system into **parasympathetic mode** (rest and digest).

Try this before bed or during the day:

Box Breathing (4-4-4-4):

- Inhale for 4 seconds
- Hold for 4 seconds
- Exhale for 4 seconds
- Hold for 4 seconds
- Repeat for 2–5 minutes

Key Takeaway: Your Hormones Thrive on Rhythm, Not Chaos

A consistent sleep-wake pattern, gentle stress management, and intentional relaxation are foundational for hormone repair—especially in your 40s and beyond. The more you support your circadian rhythm, the more your hormones will thank you.

Next, we'll dive into **Chapter 11: Natural Detox for Endocrine Support**—where you'll learn how to support your liver, lymph, and gut to safely eliminate excess hormones and toxins that disrupt your system.

Let's clear something up right away: **detoxing** isn't about juice cleanses, starvation, or expensive gimmicks. Your body already *has* a detox system—and it's working 24/7.

But here's the problem: modern life exposes you to more toxins than ever before. From pesticides and plastics to processed food and air pollution, your body is constantly under chemical stress. Over time, this toxic load can overwhelm your detox systems—especially your **liver, gut, kidneys, lymph, and skin**—and throw your hormones into chaos.

This chapter is all about how to support your natural detox pathways, so your body can eliminate **excess estrogen, cortisol, synthetic chemicals, and endocrine disruptors** more efficiently—keeping your hormones happy and balanced.

Why Detoxing Matters for Hormone Health

When your body can't properly detox hormones and toxins, they **build up** and create imbalance. Here's what that looks like:

- **Estrogen dominance** (causing PMS, heavy periods, mood swings, weight gain)
- **Thyroid disruption** (from fluoride, chlorine, BPA, and mercury)
- **Low testosterone** (due to estrogen buildup and poor liver detox)
- **Insulin resistance** (from chronic inflammation and toxic overload)

- **Cortisol dysfunction** (when your body is overwhelmed and inflamed)

The good news? You can support these detox processes gently and naturally—without harsh cleanses or deprivation.

Your Main Detox Organs (and How They Work)

1. **Liver** – filters hormones, toxins, medications, and metabolizes estrogen
2. **Gut** – eliminates waste and old hormones through bowel movements
3. **Kidneys** – flush out water-soluble toxins through urine
4. **Lymphatic system** – transports waste and immune cells through the body
5. **Skin** – eliminates toxins via sweat

When these systems are sluggish, hormones get recycled and reabsorbed—leading to symptoms.

Signs You May Need Hormone-Supportive Detox

- Bloating or constipation
- Fatigue or brain fog
- PMS or heavy periods
- Stubborn belly fat
- Skin issues (acne, eczema, dullness)
- Mood swings or irritability

- Puffy face or swollen lymph nodes
- Sensitivity to smells or chemicals

7 Ways to Support Natural Detox for Hormonal Balance

1. Eat Liver-Loving Foods Daily

Your liver is your main detox organ. It processes old hormones (especially estrogen) and neutralizes toxins so they can be eliminated through the gut and urine.

Top liver-supporting foods:

- Cruciferous vegetables (broccoli, kale, cabbage, Brussels sprouts)
- Beets and carrots (support bile flow and phase 2 detox)
- Lemon water (stimulates liver enzymes)
- Garlic and onions (contain sulfur to support detox pathways)
- Artichokes, dandelion greens, and turmeric

Pro tip: Aim for 2–3 servings of cruciferous veggies every day.

2. Prioritize Daily Bowel Movements

If you're not pooping every day, excess estrogen and toxins sit in your gut and get reabsorbed. Regular elimination is crucial.

Support strategies:

- Eat 25–35g of fiber daily (flaxseed, chia, lentils, berries, leafy greens)

- Stay hydrated (at least half your body weight in ounces of water)
- Take magnesium citrate or natural laxatives if needed short-term
- Move your body daily to support motility

3. Hydrate for Kidney Detox

Your kidneys filter blood and eliminate water-soluble toxins through urine. They need fluids to function properly.

Support strategies:

- Drink clean, filtered water (avoid tap if contaminated)
- Add a pinch of mineral-rich sea salt to water for better absorption
- Include herbal teas that support kidneys: nettle, dandelion leaf, parsley

Pro tip: Start your day with 16 oz. of lemon water to flush toxins.

4. Minimize Toxin Exposure

Reduce the toxic load coming in, so your body can focus on what's already inside.

Avoid these common endocrine disruptors:

- BPA (in plastics and canned foods)
- Phthalates (in fragrances, personal care)
- Parabens (in lotions, shampoos)

- Pesticides (on non-organic produce)
- Heavy metals (from seafood, cookware, tap water)

Simple swaps:

- Use glass or stainless steel containers
- Switch to natural cleaning products
- Choose EWG-verified personal care items
- Eat organic when possible—especially the Dirty Dozen

5. Sweat It Out

Your skin is your largest detox organ—and sweat helps release toxins stored in fat and tissue.

Ways to sweat intentionally:

- Exercise (especially strength training + cardio)
- Infrared sauna or hot Epsom salt baths
- Hot yoga or sauna blankets
- Dry brushing to stimulate lymph flow

6. Support Your Lymphatic System

Your lymph moves waste, immune cells, and fluids—but it doesn't have a pump. You have to *move it.*

Simple lymph-boosting practices:

- Dry brushing (before showers)
- Rebounding (mini trampoline)

- Whole Body Vibration Plates
- Walking, stretching, yoga
- Staying hydrated
- Contrast showers (alternating hot/cold water)

7. Consider Detox-Supportive Supplements

Helpful additions (not replacements for real food):

Supplement	Benefits
Milk Thistle	Supports liver repair and regeneration
Dandelion Root	Enhances bile flow and digestion
NAC (N-Acetyl Cysteine)	Precursor to glutathione, your body's master antioxidant
DIM (Diindolylmethane)	Supports estrogen metabolism (from cruciferous veggies)
Calcium-D-Glucarate	Aids in estrogen detox and liver clearance
Probiotics	Keeps gut microbiome healthy for proper elimination

Note: Always consult with a practitioner before adding new supplements—especially if you're on medications or managing chronic conditions.

Sample "Detox Day" for Hormone Support

Morning:

- Lemon water + dry brushing
- Breakfast: Protein smoothie with flaxseed, spinach, frozen berries, and collagen
- Milk thistle or liver support tea

Midday:

- Lunch: Quinoa bowl with roasted beets, broccoli, greens, and tahini-lemon dressing
- Herbal tea with dandelion or nettle

Evening:

- Dinner: Wild salmon with sautéed kale and garlic, side of sweet potatoes
- Light walk or Epsom salt bath
- Calming tea (chamomile + reishi) before bed

Key Takeaway: Detox Isn't a Trend—It's a Daily Practice

When your detox systems are strong, your hormones stay in harmony. You don't need a 7-day cleanse—you need *sustainable support* for your liver, gut, and lymphatic system every single day.

Clear the overload, and your body will do the rest.

Up next: **Chapter 12 – Exercise That Supports (Not Wrecks) Hormones**, where we'll talk about how to move your body in ways that enhance hormone production and reduce stress instead of making things worse.

When it comes to exercise and hormone health, the saying *"more is not always better"* couldn't be more true—especially after 40.

Yes, movement is essential for balancing hormones, boosting energy, and improving mood. But if you're doing the **wrong kind of exercise**—too intense, too frequent, or without enough recovery—you could be making your hormonal imbalance worse.

This chapter is all about learning how to move smarter—not harder—to **support hormone health, reduce stress, and optimize your metabolism** without burning out your adrenals or crashing your energy.

The Hormone–Exercise Connection

Exercise affects nearly every major hormone in your body:

Hormone	Exercise Effect
Cortisol	Spikes during intense exercise—good in short bursts, bad when overdone
Insulin	Becomes more efficient—exercise increases sensitivity
Testosterone	Increases with strength training and adequate rest
Estrogen	Stabilizes with movement and fat loss (in women)
Progesterone	Can drop if cortisol is too high

Hormone	Exercise Effect
Growth Hormone	Boosted with strength and high-intensity interval training
Thyroid Hormones	Optimized with moderate, consistent movement

The key? **Finding the right balance between challenge and recovery**.

Signs You're Overdoing It

Many people—especially those trying to lose weight or "get toned"—unintentionally overtrain. But too much high-intensity exercise can flood your system with cortisol and backfire.

Warning signs:

- Feeling exhausted after workouts
- Trouble sleeping or waking at 3 a.m.
- Craving sugar or carbs post-exercise
- Stalled weight loss despite more effort
- Increased anxiety, mood swings, or irritability
- Loss of menstrual cycle (in women)
- Plateauing in strength or progress

Best Types of Exercise for Hormone Balance

1. Strength Training (2–4x per week)

This is the #1 best form of exercise for hormone health in both men and women over 40.

Benefits:

- Boosts testosterone, growth hormone, and insulin sensitivity
- Preserves lean muscle and bone density
- Improves mood and metabolism

How to do it:

- Focus on full-body workouts: squats, lunges, deadlifts, push-ups, rows
- Use dumbbells, kettle bells, resistance bands, or body weight
- Rest 48 hours between sessions per muscle group
- Keep sessions short (30–45 minutes)

2. Walking and Low-Intensity Cardio (Daily or 4–6x/week)

Never underestimate the power of walking—especially for reducing cortisol and improving insulin response.

Benefits:

- Lowers stress hormones
- Improves fat metabolism
- Supports lymphatic movement and digestion

How to do it:

- Aim for 7,000–10,000 steps per day

- Use a walking desk, take post-meal walks, or go outside after dinner
- Try walking meditations or podcasts to multitask mentally

3. Yoga, Pilates, and Mobility Work (2–3x per week)

Gentle movement nourishes your nervous system and reduces inflammation.

Benefits:

- Enhances flexibility, joint health, and circulation
- Balances the nervous system (reducing fight-or-flight response)
- Improves breath control and emotional resilience

How to do it:

- Include 10–20 minutes of stretching on rest days or after workouts
- Try restorative or yin yoga in the evening for sleep support
- Mix in Pilates or mobility drills to improve posture and joint stability

4. HIIT (High-Intensity Interval Training) – Use with Caution (1–2x per week MAX)

HIIT can be powerful, but over 40, it must be used strategically.

Benefits:

- Increases growth hormone and cardiovascular fitness
- Torches calories in a short amount of time

The risk:

- Overdoing it raises cortisol, suppresses thyroid, and can stall fat loss

How to do it right:

- Limit to 15–25 minutes per session
- Space 2–3 days apart
- Prioritize recovery: sleep, hydration, and fueling

Movement & Hormone Tips by Goal

Goal	Best Approach
Balance Cortisol	Daily walks, restorative yoga, short strength sessions
Boost Testosterone	Strength training, sprints (with rest), adequate sleep
Improve Insulin Sensitivity	Walking after meals, full-body resistance workouts
Reduce Estrogen Dominance	Sweating regularly, detox support, moderate intensity cardio
Support Thyroid	Gentle strength + low-impact cardio, no overtraining

Goal	Best Approach
Menopause Transition	Mobility work, short strength + walks, breath-based yoga

Create Your Hormone-Healthy Weekly Movement Plan

Here's a sample balanced schedule:

Monday – Full-body strength training (30–40 min)
Tuesday – 30–45 min walk + 15 min yoga/stretch
Wednesday – Active recovery: light movement or mobility
Thursday – Full-body strength or Pilates
Friday – Restorative yoga or walk
Saturday – Optional HIIT or hike (short and energizing)
Sunday – Rest or gentle walk + Epsom salt bath

Don't Forget to Fuel Your Workouts

Eating around your workouts helps protect your muscles and hormones:

- **Before workout:** small protein-rich snack or amino acid drinks if needed (e.g., boiled eggs, protein shake)
- **After workout:** protein + carbs within 30–60 minutes (e.g., smoothie, chicken + sweet potato)
- **Hydrate well:** add electrolytes to water if sweating a lot

Key Takeaway: Train for Balance, Not Burnout

In your 40s and beyond, your goal isn't punishment—it's **hormonal harmony**. The right exercise makes you feel strong, stable, energized, and clear-headed—not depleted or anxious.

Train smart. Rest often. And move your body in a way that supports your hormones for the long haul.

Next up is **Chapter 13: Supplements That Actually Work**, where we'll break down which vitamins, minerals, and herbs are worth taking to support hormone balance—without wasting your money.

Chapter 13: Supplements That Actually Work for Hormonal Balance

Let's face it—there are **a lot** of supplements out there. Walk down the vitamin aisle or scroll through your social media feed and you'll be bombarded with promises of "hormone balance in a bottle."

But here's the truth: **supplements should support your foundation, not replace it.** If you're not sleeping well, eating real food, managing stress, and moving your body, no supplement will magically fix your hormones.

That said, the **right supplements** can fill nutritional gaps, restore depleted reserves, and gently nudge your body back into balance—especially after 40, when your needs change.

This chapter cuts through the noise and focuses on **evidence-based, effective, and safe** supplements that can truly support hormonal health—for both women and men.

How to Supplement Smart

Before we dive in, here are a few golden rules:

- **Get tested when possible** (especially for vitamin D, thyroid, iron, sex hormones, and cortisol)
- **Choose high-quality brands** with third-party testing and no artificial fillers
- **Start low and go slow**—introduce one supplement at a time to track how you feel
- **Cycle your supplements** every few months if you're taking them long-term

- **Food comes first**—supplements are meant to *supplement*, not substitute

Essential Supplements for Everyone Over 40

These core nutrients support overall hormone health, energy, brain function, and stress resilience.

1. Magnesium (Glycinate or Citrate)

Benefits:

- Calms the nervous system, improves sleep, reduces PMS
- Supports over 300 enzymatic functions, including hormone metabolism
- Eases anxiety, constipation, and muscle tension

Suggested dose: 300–400 mg per day (split doses if needed)
Best forms: magnesium glycinate (calming), citrate (for regularity)

2. Vitamin D3 + K2

Benefits:

- Supports estrogen, testosterone, mood, immunity, and bone health
- Often deficient in adults over 40
- Works synergistically with calcium and magnesium

Suggested dose: 2,000–5,000 IU daily with fat-containing meal
Always pair with K2 for calcium metabolism

3. Omega-3 Fatty Acids (Fish Oil)

Benefits:

- Reduces inflammation and supports hormone production
- Boosts brain health, mood, skin, and metabolism
- Helps regulate insulin and cortisol

Suggested dose: 1,000–2,000 mg EPA/DHA per day
Choose triglyceride-form, molecularly distilled fish oil or algae-based for plant-based option

4. B-Complex Vitamins

Benefits:

- Vital for adrenal function, mood, energy, and detoxification
- Supports estrogen and progesterone metabolism
- Helps your body cope with stress

Suggested dose: As directed on a full-spectrum B-complex
Look for methylated forms (e.g., methyl-B12, methylfolate)

5. Probiotics

Benefits:

- Balances gut microbiome, essential for estrogen and cortisol regulation
- Improves digestion, immune function, and mood
- Aids in hormone detox through the estrobolome

Suggested dose: 10–50 billion CFU daily
Look for strains like Lactobacillus and Bifidobacterium

Targeted Supplements for Women

1. Vitex (Chasteberry)

Best for: Low progesterone, irregular cycles, PMS, perimenopause
How it works: Supports luteal phase and balances estrogen-to-progesterone ratio
Caution: Best taken in the morning; do not use if on hormonal birth control

2. DIM (Diindolylmethane)

Best for: Estrogen dominance, heavy periods, fibroids, PMS
How it works: Supports healthy estrogen metabolism through the liver
Caution: Should be paired with liver support (e.g., milk thistle, B vitamins)

3. Evening Primrose Oil

Best for: Hormonal acne, breast tenderness, dry skin, PMS
How it works: Provides GLA (gamma-linolenic acid), a healthy omega-6 fatty acid
Suggested dose: 500–1,300 mg daily with food

4. Maca Root

Best for: Fatigue, low libido, mood swings, menopause transition
How it works: Acts as an adaptogen to support energy and endocrine function
Forms: Gelatinized powder or capsules—start with 500–1,000 mg daily

Targeted Supplements for Men

1. Zinc

Best for: Testosterone support, immune function, prostate health
How it works: Essential cofactor in testosterone production and sperm health
Suggested dose: 15–30 mg daily (not to exceed 50 mg)

2. DHEA *(use with lab guidance)*

Best for: Fatigue, low testosterone, burnout, low libido
How it works: Precursor hormone for estrogen and testosterone
Caution: Get your levels tested—too much can cause side effects

3. Tribulus Terrestris

Best for: Libido, stamina, testosterone support
How it works: Natural herb shown to enhance male sexual function and vitality
Suggested dose: Follow product label; cycle 6–8 weeks on, 2 weeks off

4. Tongkat Ali

Best for: Testosterone production, stress reduction, muscle maintenance
How it works: Helps release bound testosterone and reduce cortisol
Suggested dose: 200–400 mg per day

Supplements to Support Stress & Adrenal Recovery

These are helpful for anyone—male or female—dealing with burnout, anxiety, poor sleep, or cortisol imbalance.

Supplement	**Supports**
Ashwagandha	Lowers cortisol, improves sleep and mood
Rhodiola Rosea	Boosts energy, stamina, and mental clarity
L-theanine	Calms anxiety without sedation
Phosphatidylserine	Helps lower nighttime cortisol
Reishi Mushroom	Supports immune and stress response

What NOT to Waste Money On

- Detox teas and flat tummy products
- "Hormone balancers" with mystery blends and no dosing transparency
- Gimmicky powders or gummies with underdosed ingredients
- Overuse of melatonin (use short-term only if needed)

Key Takeaway: Supplements Can Be a Game-Changer—If You Use Them Wisely

The right supplements can give your body the nudge it needs to rebalance naturally—but only when paired with good sleep, food, movement, and stress support.

Listen to your body. Use testing where possible. And remember: **you're not fixing a problem—you're supporting a system.**

Next up: **Chapter 14 – Creating a Hormone-Smart Daily Routine**, where we'll bring everything together into a practical, easy-to-follow day designed to help you thrive.

So, you've learned what your hormones are, how they work, what throws them off, and how to support them. Now it's time to bring it all together.

Hormonal harmony doesn't happen from one thing you do once—it happens from what you do consistently.

A daily routine that supports your hormones is like laying down train tracks for your body to run smoothly on. The more consistent your routine, the more balanced and energized you'll feel—mentally, physically, and emotionally.

This chapter helps you **build your own hormone-smart day** with practical habits that work in real life, even if you're busy, stressed, or just getting started.

Why Routines Matter for Hormones

Your body *loves* rhythm. It's designed to follow natural patterns—like the rising and setting of the sun, the sleep-wake cycle, and your monthly hormonal cycle (if you're menstruating).

When you follow a consistent routine:

- **Cortisol stabilizes** (less stress and belly fat)
- **Insulin levels even out** (better energy and metabolism)
- **Sleep improves** (more melatonin and growth hormone)
- **Sex hormones rebalance** (less PMS, more libido, improved mood)

Small, simple habits performed regularly can profoundly affect how you feel.

Morning Routine: Set the Tone for the Day

1. Get Sunlight Within 30 Minutes of Waking

Supports cortisol rhythm, boosts mood, and improves sleep later that night

Try: A 10-minute walk outside or sitting by a sunny window

2. Drink 16–20 oz. of Water Before Coffee

Rehydrates cells, flushes toxins, supports digestion

Add lemon or a pinch of sea salt for extra minerals

3. Eat a Hormone-Friendly Breakfast

Includes protein, healthy fats, and fiber

Example: Eggs, avocado, and spinach OR a protein smoothie with flax and berries

4. Move Your Body—Even Briefly

Morning movement improves blood sugar and mood

Try: A brisk 10-minute walk, mobility flow, or strength workout

5. Take Your Foundational Supplements

Magnesium, omega-3s, vitamin D, B-complex, or adaptogens

Consistency is key—set a reminder or leave them out where you'll see them

Midday Routine: Balance Blood Sugar + Calm the Nervous System

1. Eat a Balanced Lunch

Aim for protein + fiber + healthy fat

Example: Salmon salad with olive oil and sweet potato

2. Step Away From Work to Eat

Eating mindfully supports digestion and reduces stress

Even 10 minutes away from screens helps

3. Go for a 10–15 Minute Walk After Lunch
Supports blood sugar and energy
This one habit dramatically improves insulin sensitivity

4. Do a Midday Stress Reset
3–5 minutes of deep breathing, stretching, or a short meditation
Try: Box breathing or alternate nostril breathing

Optional Supplements:

- Rhodiola or holy basil if energy is low
- Digestive enzymes if digestion is sluggish

Evening Routine: Wind Down + Support Detox + Sleep

1. Eat Dinner 2–3 Hours Before Bed
Gives your body time to digest and reduces blood sugar spikes overnight
Aim for lean protein + veggies + complex carbs (like quinoa or sweet potatoes)

2. Limit Blue Light Exposure After Sunset
Too much screen time suppresses melatonin
Use blue light blockers, switch to warm lighting, or read a book instead

3. Take a Calming Supplement or Tea
Magnesium glycinate, reishi, L-theanine, or chamomile tea
Helps your nervous system unwind and improves sleep quality

4. Epsom Salt Bath or Gentle Stretching
Supports detox, lowers cortisol, and calms the mind
Add lavender essential oil or soft music for extra relaxation

5. Bedtime by 10–10:30 PM
Sleep before midnight is more restorative and supports hormone

repair
Keep your room cool, dark, and screen-free

Mindset & Consistency Tips

- **Pick 3 habits to start with.** Don't try to do it all at once.
- **Stack habits together.** Take your supplements with breakfast. Do breathwork while your tea steeps.
- **Track how you feel.** Use a simple journal or app to note energy, mood, sleep, cycle symptoms, or digestion.
- **Be flexible, not perfect.** It's not about rigidity—it's about rhythm.

Your Hormone-Smart Daily Checklist

Morning:

- ☐ Sunlight exposure
- ☐ Hydration
- ☐ Protein-rich breakfast
- ☐ Movement
- ☐ Foundational supplements

Midday:

- ☐ Balanced lunch
- ☐ Walk after eating
- ☐ Stress break / breathwork

- ☐ Support digestion (if needed)

Evening:

- ☐ Light dinner, early
- ☐ Wind-down routine
- ☐ Magnesium or calming tea
- ☐ Tech off, lights down
- ☐ Sleep by 10:30 PM

Key Takeaway: Your Routine is Your Medicine

You don't need to overhaul your life—you need to align with your body's natural rhythm. When you eat, move, rest, and recover in sync with your hormones, everything gets easier: energy improves, cycles regulate, mood lifts, and your body feels *safe* to heal.

Up next: **Chapter 15 – When to Get Tested & What to Ask For**, where we'll walk through the most important hormone-related tests, what your results really mean, and how to advocate for yourself with healthcare providers.

Sometimes, the best way to take control of your hormone health is to stop guessing and **start testing**.

Your symptoms—fatigue, mood swings, weight gain, low libido, poor sleep—are real. But to know *what's really going on* under the surface, you need data. Testing gives you insight, clarity, and a targeted path forward. It's not about labels—it's about empowerment.

In this chapter, you'll learn **what hormone-related tests to ask for, when to test, how to interpret your results**, and how to advocate for yourself with your healthcare provider—especially if you feel like you're being dismissed.

Why Testing Matters

- Confirms (or rules out) hormone imbalances
- Provides a baseline to track your progress over time
- Helps avoid unnecessary medications or supplements
- Reveals hidden patterns, like estrogen dominance or adrenal fatigue
- Ensures you're targeting the *right* issue—not chasing symptoms

When to Get Tested

You should consider hormone testing if you're experiencing:

- Chronic fatigue despite rest

- Unexplained weight gain or weight loss resistance
- Irregular or heavy periods
- Hair thinning or skin changes
- Low sex drive or erectile dysfunction
- Mood issues: anxiety, depression, irritability
- Brain fog or poor memory
- Hot flashes, night sweats, or sleep problems
- PMS, PCOS, or perimenopausal symptoms
- Difficulty building muscle or recovering from workouts

Pro tip: Track your symptoms for 1–2 months beforehand. Use a simple notebook or hormone health app. This makes your case stronger when speaking to your doctor.

Top Hormone Labs to Request (for Men & Women)

Sex Hormones

Test	Why it Matters
Estrogen (Estradiol, E2)	High = estrogen dominance, Low = menopausal symptoms
Progesterone	Low = anxiety, sleep issues, PMS, fertility struggles
Testosterone (Total & Free)	Low = fatigue, low libido, poor recovery in men *and* women

Test	Why it Matters
DHEA-S	Precursor to estrogen/testosterone; indicator of adrenal health
SHBG (Sex Hormone Binding Globulin)	High = less available testosterone/estrogen

Adrenal Function

Test	Why it Matters
Cortisol (4-point saliva or DUTCH test)	Reveals stress hormone rhythm, adrenal fatigue, burnout
ACTH	Stimulates cortisol production—low = adrenal insufficiency

Best cortisol tests: Saliva or urine (DUTCH test). A single blood cortisol draw often misses the full picture.

Thyroid Function

Test	Why it Matters
TSH	Basic screening (but not enough alone!)
Free T3 & Free T4	Show how well your thyroid is actually functioning
Reverse T3	High = stress, inflammation, low conversion

Test	Why it Matters
Thyroid Antibodies (TPO, TgAb)	Rule out autoimmune thyroid disease (Hashimoto's)

Metabolic & Blood Sugar Markers

Test	Why it Matters
Fasting Insulin	Early marker of insulin resistance
Fasting Glucose	Should be between 75–90 for optimal hormone balance
HbA1c	3-month average blood sugar—important for weight, fertility
Lipid Panel	Hormones are made from cholesterol—too low isn't ideal

Advanced Testing Options (if available):

- **DUTCH Complete Test** (urine): Gold standard for sex hormones, cortisol, DHEA, melatonin
- **GI MAP or GI Effects (stool):** Gut health impacts estrogen clearance and cortisol levels
- **Hair Tissue Mineral Analysis (HTMA):** Shows mineral deficiencies that impact thyroid, adrenals, and metabolism

When to Test in Your Cycle (Women)

Timing is everything—especially if you're still menstruating.

Hormone	Best Time to Test
Progesterone	Days 19–21 of a 28-day cycle (mid-luteal phase)
Estradiol	Day 3 of cycle (early follicular phase)
Testosterone/DHEA	Day 3 or any time if cycle is irregular

If you're **postmenopausal**, you can test anytime—but track symptoms and context.

How to Advocate for Yourself

Many people are dismissed with phrases like:

- "Your labs are normal."
- "It's just aging."
- "You're probably just stressed."

Here's how to respond with confidence:

1. Be informed. Bring a symptom tracker and list of specific tests you want.
2. Be direct. Say: *"I want to investigate possible hormone imbalance, and I'm looking for a comprehensive panel."*
3. Be persistent. If your provider says "no," ask *why*. Then consider seeking a functional or integrative medicine practitioner.
4. Consider private labs. Many companies now offer at-home hormone testing without a doctor's order.

What If Your Tests Come Back "Normal"—But You Don't Feel Normal?

This is **very common.** Lab ranges are based on the average population—not optimal wellness. You may fall within the "normal" range but still have suboptimal levels for your body.

Here's where a skilled practitioner can make a huge difference. Look for one who:

- Listens to your symptoms, not just your labs
- Considers optimal ranges, not just reference ranges
- Looks at how hormones interact—not just individual markers

Key Takeaway: You Deserve to Know What's Really Going On

Testing is a powerful tool—not a diagnosis, but a *map.* It helps you identify root causes, measure progress, and make smart, targeted choices for your health.

You're not crazy. You're not lazy. If you feel "off," there's a reason—and the right tests can help you find it.

Up next: **Chapter 16 – Sample 7-Day Hormone Reset Plan**, where you'll get a complete food, movement, and lifestyle plan to kickstart your hormone healing journey naturally.

By now, you've learned what hormones do, how they become imbalanced, and how lifestyle habits can either restore or wreck your internal harmony. But putting it all into practice can feel overwhelming.

That's why this chapter gives you a **done-for-you, 7-day hormone reset plan**—a simple, flexible routine designed to calm inflammation, support detox, balance blood sugar, and gently bring your hormones back into alignment.

This isn't a crash diet or strict cleanse. It's a foundation for feeling better—fast.

Goals of This Reset Plan

- Stabilize cortisol and blood sugar
- Support liver detox (especially for estrogen and toxins)
- Boost progesterone and testosterone naturally
- Calm the nervous system
- Improve energy, digestion, mood, and sleep

How to Use This Plan

- Follow for 7 days straight, or use as a flexible guideline.
- Hydrate throughout the day—aim for half your body weight in ounces of clean water.
- Take your foundational supplements: magnesium, omega-3s, vitamin D, B-complex.

- Get 7–9 hours of quality sleep per night.
- Swap meals as needed, but stick to the principles.
- Most importantly—listen to your body.

Your Daily Hormone Reset Template

Morning Routine

- Wake up and get sunlight for 10–20 min
- Drink warm lemon water with a pinch of sea salt
- Optional: Breathwork or journaling (5–10 min)
- Protein-rich breakfast within 60 minutes of waking
- **Meals (3 balanced meals per day + optional snack)**
  Each meal should include:

- Protein (20–30g)
- Healthy fats (avocado, olive oil, seeds, etc.)
- Fiber (veggies, flax, chia, beans, etc.)
- Low-glycemic carbs (quinoa, sweet potato, berries, etc.)

Movement

- 20–30 min walk daily (especially post-meal)
- 2–3 strength or mobility sessions per week
- Restorative yoga or stretching in the evening

Evening Routine

- Herbal tea (chamomile, reishi, lemon balm)
- Epsom salt bath or gentle stretching
- Sleep by 10:30 p.m. in a cool, dark room

7-Day Hormone Reset Plan

DAY 1: Liver Love + Gentle Movement

Breakfast: Scrambled eggs with spinach and avocado
Lunch: Lentil and roasted veggie bowl with tahini dressing
Dinner: Grilled salmon, sweet potato mash, steamed broccoli
Snack: Chia pudding with berries and cinnamon
Movement: 30-min walk + light yoga
Self-care: Dry brushing + Epsom salt bath

DAY 2: Gut Reset + Stress Relief

Breakfast: Protein smoothie (protein powder, flaxseed, almond butter, greens, berries)
Lunch: Chicken + kale salad with olive oil, beets, and pumpkin seeds
Dinner: Turkey lettuce wraps with cucumber, carrots, and cashew-lime sauce
Snack: Handful of walnuts and herbal tea
Movement: Walk after lunch + 10-min stretch
Self-care: Guided breathwork or meditation

DAY 3: Estrogen Detox Focus

Breakfast: Oatmeal with ground flax, chia seeds, and blueberries
Lunch: Quinoa + roasted Brussels sprouts, red cabbage, and lemon tahini
Dinner: Grass-fed beef stir-fry with broccoli, mushrooms, and ginger
Snack: Apple slices with almond butter
Movement: Strength training (30 mins)
Self-care: Detox tea + magnesium supplement before bed

DAY 4: Blood Sugar Balance + Focus

Breakfast: Veggie omelet with side of sauerkraut
Lunch: Tuna salad-stuffed avocado with side of carrots and hummus
Dinner: Baked cod, garlic sautéed kale, and roasted carrots
Snack: Coconut yogurt with cinnamon and seeds
Movement: 20-min walk + rebounding or stretching
Self-care: Journaling + screen-free hour before bed

DAY 5: Calm and Restore

Breakfast: Protein smoothie with maca and cinnamon
Lunch: Chickpea curry with basmati rice and cilantro
Dinner: Lemon herb chicken, sautéed spinach, and sweet potato
Snack: Cucumber slices and guacamole
Movement: Yoga or Pilates (30 min)
Self-care: Epsom bath + deep breathing before sleep

DAY 6: Testosterone & Metabolism Boost

Breakfast: Turkey sausage, eggs, and sautéed kale
Lunch: Bison or turkey burger (no bun) with roasted zucchini and avocado

Dinner: Grilled shrimp, quinoa, and roasted asparagus
Snack: Boiled eggs + sliced bell pepper
Movement: Strength training (35–40 min full-body)
Self-care: Cold shower or contrast hydrotherapy

DAY 7: Integration + Reflection

Breakfast: Smoothie bowl with greens, chia, flax, and berries
Lunch: Detox veggie soup with lentils and sweet potatoes
Dinner: Wild-caught salmon sushi bowl with rice, seaweed, avocado, and cucumber
Snack: Herbal tea + 1 square of 85% dark chocolate
Movement: Nature walk or hiking
Self-care: Reflect + journal on what you learned and how you feel

Reflection Questions

At the end of the 7 days, ask yourself:

- How's my energy?
- Am I sleeping better?
- Is my mood more stable?
- Has my digestion improved?
- What habits made the biggest impact?
- What do I want to continue long-term?

What's Next?

You can repeat this reset monthly, or use it anytime your hormones feel "off." Better yet—take what worked and **build it into your new normal.**

You're not just resetting your hormones—you're building **a lifestyle that supports your body every day.**

Next up is **Chapter 17: Resources & Recommended Products**, where we'll share trusted tools, apps, supplements, and wellness brands to support your hormone journey.

You've built a foundation of knowledge, started aligning your habits with your hormonal health, and even completed a 7-day hormone reset. Now it's time to **equip yourself with the right tools** to support this journey long-term.

This chapter is your go-to guide for **trusted products, tools, books, apps, and wellness brands** that support hormone health naturally. Whether you're looking for supplements, non-toxic skincare, lab tests, or educational resources—you'll find it all here.

Recommended At-Home Hormone & Health Testing

These options give you access to hormone data without needing a doctor's order (though it's always best to interpret results with a qualified provider).

1. DUTCH Test (Precision Analytical)

- In-depth urine test for sex hormones, cortisol, melatonin, and metabolites
- Excellent for evaluating estrogen dominance, adrenal fatigue, and hormone detox
- Website: www.dutchtest.com

2. Everlywell

- At-home kits for thyroid, cortisol, testosterone, and food sensitivities
- Easy-to-understand reports
- Website: www.everlywell.com

3. LetsGetChecked

- Discreet home testing for testosterone, female hormones, thyroid, and more
- CLIA-certified labs
- Website: www.letsgetchecked.com

Top-Quality Supplement Brands (Hormone-Friendly)

Always choose brands with **third-party testing, no artificial fillers**, and transparent sourcing.

Brand	What They're Great For
Pure Encapsulations	Clean, hypoallergenic supplements (B-complex, magnesium)
Thorne Research	High-quality hormone and liver support (DIM, DHEA, Zinc)
Designs for Health	Comprehensive wellness line, including hormone balancing kits
Seeking Health	Methylated vitamins, prenatal support, and adrenal blends
Vital Proteins	Clean collagen peptides for gut, skin, and joint support
Gaia Herbs	Herbal tinctures and adaptogens (ashwagandha, reishi, maca)
MegaFood	Whole food-based multis and women's formulas

Tip: Always check for gluten, soy, dairy, and artificial sweeteners if you're sensitive.

Non-Toxic Skincare & Beauty Brands

What goes **on your body** is just as important as what goes **in it**—especially for hormone balance. Many conventional products contain endocrine disruptors like parabens, phthalates, and synthetic fragrances.

Recommended brands:

- **Primally Pure** – Tallow-based creams, deodorants, and oils
- **Beautycounter** – EWG-verified, clean makeup and skincare
- **True Botanicals** – Hormone-safe anti-aging serums and cleansers
- **Native** – Aluminum-free deodorant with clean ingredients
- **Alaffia** – Affordable and ethically-sourced body care
- **Branch Basics** – Non-toxic cleaning products for home and laundry

Books Worth Reading on Hormonal Health

- **"The Hormone Cure" by Dr. Sara Gottfried**
  A functional medicine approach to balancing hormones naturally.

- **"In the FLO" by Alisa Vitti**
  Cycle syncing for women—eat, move, and work in alignment with your hormonal phases.

- **"Why Zebras Don't Get Ulcers" by Robert Sapolsky**
  A deep dive into stress, cortisol, and how it affects the body and brain.

- **"Roar" by Dr. Stacy Sims**
  Training and nutrition for women over 40, especially athletes or active individuals.

- **"Adrenal Transformation Protocol" by Dr. Izabella Wentz**
  A practical guide to recovering from stress, burnout, and adrenal dysfunction.

Apps for Tracking and Support

App	**Use It For**
MyFlo	Track your cycle, get phase-specific tips
Clue	Hormone and period tracking for women
Oura Ring App	Sleep, HRV, and cycle readiness tracking
Chronometer	Nutrition tracking with micronutrient detail
Insight Timer	Guided breathwork, meditation, and stress relief
Mighty Health	Hormone-focused wellness programs for 40+

Bonus Tools to Support Your Journey

- **Dry Brush** – Stimulates lymphatic system and detox pathways
- **Blue Light Blocking Glasses** – Protect melatonin at night
- **Epsom Salt (Magnesium Sulfate)** – Supports detox and relaxation
- **Infrared Sauna Blanket or Mat** – Boosts circulation and hormone detox
- **Castor Oil Packs** – Liver and lymph support, especially during PMS or perimenopause
- **Collagen Protein Powder** – Gut, skin, and joint support, especially post-menopause

Practitioner Types to Look For

If you're ready to get more personalized help, these professionals specialize in hormonal health:

- **Functional Medicine Doctors**
- **Naturopathic Doctors (NDs)**
- **Integrative Health Practitioners**
- **Nutritional Therapy Practitioners (NTPs)**
- **Hormone Health Coaches (certified)**
- **Women's Health Nurse Practitioners (WHNPs)**

Tip: Use directories like IFM.org (Institute for Functional Medicine) or AANP.org to find a provider near you.

Key Takeaway: Equip Your Environment for Success

The more you reduce friction and surround yourself with supportive tools and products, the easier it becomes to live in alignment with your hormones.

You don't need to buy everything at once. Just start with one swap, one upgrade, or one tool that makes you feel more in control—and build from there.

Up next is **Chapter 18: Conclusion – Thriving Naturally in Your 40s and Beyond**, where we'll wrap everything up with encouragement, clarity, and your next best steps.

Chapter 18: Conclusion – Thriving Naturally in Your 40s and Beyond

You've made it to the end of this guide—but truly, this is just the beginning.

The journey through your 40s, 50s, and beyond isn't about fighting your body. It's about *reconnecting* with it.

Your hormones are not the enemy. They're your body's messengers—alerting you when something's off and guiding you toward what it needs most: nourishment, rest, balance, and care.

This chapter is your invitation to take everything you've learned and apply it—not with perfection, but with intention.

What You've Gained

Over the past 18 chapters, you've uncovered the foundations of natural hormone health:

- **Understanding** how hormones like estrogen, progesterone, testosterone, cortisol, insulin, and thyroid hormones work
- **Recognizing** the signs of imbalance (and knowing they're not "just aging")
- **Learning** how stress, sleep, nutrition, and toxins impact your endocrine system
- **Discovering** powerful tools—from adaptogens and detox practices to sleep routines and strength training
- **Building** a daily rhythm that supports your mind, metabolism, and mood

This is the work that *prevents disease, restores vitality, and empowers longevity*.

This Isn't About Perfect Health—It's About Empowered Health

You will have off days. You'll skip workouts. You'll eat cake at the party. You'll forget your supplements.

And that's okay.

The goal is not perfection. It's **alignment**—a lifestyle that makes your body feel safe, supported, and loved.

Because when your hormones feel safe, your energy improves. Your mind clears. Your weight stabilizes. Your skin glows. Your joy returns.

This isn't a trend. This is your *biology working for you*, not against you.

Your Next Best Steps

Here's how to keep the momentum going:

Pick 2–3 core habits you loved from the 7-day reset and make them part of your daily routine.
Get tested, if you haven't already, and track your progress with real data.
Build your hormone support system—whether that's a journal, a coach, or a group of friends on the same journey.
Revisit this guide when life throws you off course. It's here as your map.
Celebrate your wins—more energy, better sleep, less pain, stronger boundaries… these are victories worth noticing.

Final Words of Encouragement

Your body isn't broken. It's brilliant.

Every symptom you've felt has been a whisper from your hormones—a call to slow down, tune in, and reset.

The best part? You've already started.

This isn't the end of your wellness story. It's a new chapter—one where you feel **more connected, more clear, and more confident** in your body than you have in years.

Let this book be your reminder:
You don't have to hustle for health.
You don't need to fear midlife.
And you're not alone.

Your hormones can work for you—not against you—when you learn how to listen.

So here's to your healing. Your energy. Your strength. Your softness. Your power.

Here's to your hormone harmony—for life.

Resources

Here's a **comprehensive list of credible resources and references** that support the information presented throughout this hormone health guidebook. These sources span medical literature, functional and integrative health experts, peer-reviewed research, and respected health organizations. While the guidebook was written in an accessible, user-friendly style, its content is rooted in evidence-based principles.

Scientific Research & Medical Journals

1. **National Institutes of Health (NIH) – PubMed**
   - Hormonal fluctuations and health in midlife
   - Research on menopause, andropause, and HPA axis dysfunction
     https://pubmed.ncbi.nlm.nih.gov
2. **The Journal of Clinical Endocrinology & Metabolism (JCEM)**
   - Age-related hormonal changes, adrenal and thyroid disorders
     https://academic.oup.com/jcem
3. **American Journal of Lifestyle Medicine**
   - Studies on the impact of diet, exercise, and stress on hormone health
     https://journals.sagepub.com/home/ajl
4. **The North American Menopause Society (NAMS)**

- Guidelines on hormone replacement, perimenopause, and symptom management https://www.menopause.org

5. **The Endocrine Society**
   - Hormone function, testing, and evidence-based treatment options https://www.endocrine.org

6. **International Journal of Environmental Research and Public Health**
   - Endocrine-disrupting chemicals (EDCs) and their impact on hormonal balance https://www.mdpi.com/journal/ijerph

---

Books by Trusted Experts

1. **The Hormone Cure** – Dr. Sara Gottfried, MD
2. **The Adrenal Thyroid Revolution** – Dr. Aviva Romm, MD
3. **In the FLO** – Alisa Vitti, Functional Nutritionist
4. **The Period Repair Manual** – Lara Briden, ND
5. **Roar** – Dr. Stacy Sims, PhD (exercise science and women's physiology)
6. **The New Rules of Menopause** – Dr. Heather Hirsch, MD
7. **Adrenal Transformation Protocol** – Dr. Izabella Wentz, PharmD

Functional & Integrative Medicine Authorities

1. **Institute for Functional Medicine (IFM)**
   https://www.ifm.org
   – Functional lab testing, lifestyle-based hormone care, adrenal support protocols

2. **Chris Kresser, MS, LAc**
   https://chriskresser.com
   – Integrative health strategies for thyroid, adrenal, gut, and hormonal wellness

3. **Dr. Mark Hyman, MD – The UltraWellness Center**
   https://drhyman.com
   – Nutrition, detox, and metabolic health for hormone repair

4. **Aviva Romm, MD – Herbalist & Yale-trained Integrative Physician**
   https://avivaromm.com
   – Women's hormone health, botanicals, and natural protocols

---

Nutritional & Supplement Resources

1. **Examine.com** – Research-based analysis of supplements and bioactives
   https://www.examine.com

2. **The Linus Pauling Institute at Oregon State University**
   – Micronutrient guides for vitamin D, B-complex, magnesium, zinc
   https://lpi.oregonstate.edu

3. **National Center for Complementary and Integrative Health (NCCIH)**
   – Evidence on adaptogens like ashwagandha, rhodiola,

and maca
https://nccih.nih.gov

Lifestyle & Wellness Apps & Tools

1. **MyFlo App** – Cycle syncing support for women
   https://myflotracker.com

2. **Clue App** – Menstrual tracking and hormonal symptom logs
   https://helloclue.com

3. **Oura Ring** – Sleep, stress, and cycle tracking
   https://ouraring.com

4. **Insight Timer** – Meditation and breathwork for cortisol regulation
   https://insighttimer.com

Toxin-Free Living & EWG Data

1. **Environmental Working Group (EWG)** – Skin Deep Database
   – Ratings for cosmetics, personal care, and cleaning products
   https://www.ewg.org/skindeep

2. **Made Safe Certified Products**
   – Certified toxin-free home and body care
   https://madesafe.org

Our Favorite Resources for Creating a Healthy Life

Our Website Contains Information about our Clinic and the services we provide. Learn more at: https://www.CockrellFamilyMedical.com

Medwave's NLT Red Light Therapy is the leader in office based medical red light therapy. Learn more at: https://medwavegroup.com

(Let them know Dr. Mike Cockrell sent you and ask about any Special Pricing Offers)

Great Life Worldwide provides some of the Highest Quality Nutritional Supplements available online. Their Clear Heart Cardiovascular product and their Get Juiced Nutritional Supplements are cutting edge supplments. Learn More at: https://www.cfmc.shop

GLP Xtreme is our cutting-edge Weight Loss Supplement for a reason. Get yours today at: https://www.cfmc.shop

Some of our favorite supplements are Magnesium Complex, Amino Acid Blend, Protein Powders, Men's Vitality and Women's Vitality. You can get access to these amazing supplements at: https://www.drmikecockrell.com/best

BTL Aesthetics is the Leader in Advanced Regenerative Technologies. To Learn More go to: https://bodybybtl.com

(Let them know Dr. Mike Cockrell sent you and ask about any Special Pricing Offers)

Softwave TRT Ortho Gold is a game-changing technology that can Reduce Joint Pain and Improve Mobility with cutting edge Shockwave Technology. Learn More at: https://softwavetrt.com/orthogold/

(Let them know Dr. Mike Cockrell sent you and ask about any Special Pricing Offers)

Made in the USA
Monee, IL
04 November 2026

67379705R00069